Mediterranean Diet Cookbook

The Best Guide for Beginners.

Enjoy Tasty Dessert with Quick, Easy and Simple Recipes.

Healthy Living with Amazing Dishes.

Salads Recipes Included.

Alexangel Kitchen

Just for Our Readers

To Thank You for Purchasing the Book, for a limited time, you can get a Special FREE BOOK from Alexangel Kitchen

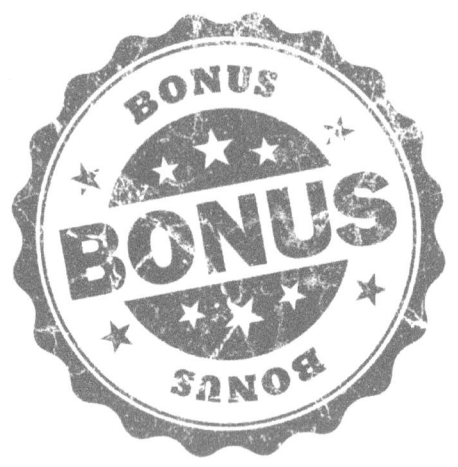

Just go to https://alexangelkitchen.com/ to download your FREE BOOK

Table of Contents

Table of Contents	4
Beans and Cucumber Salad	11
Tomato and Avocado Salad	13
Arugula Salad	14
Chickpea Salad	17
Chopped Israeli Mediterranean Pasta Salad	19
Feta Tomato Salad	21
Greek Pasta Salad	23
Watermelon Salad	25
Orange Celery Salad	28
Roasted Broccoli Salad	30
Tomato Salad	33
Feta Beet Salad	34
Cauliflower & Tomato Salad	34
Tahini Spinach	37
Pilaf with Cream Cheese	39
Easy Spaghetti Squash	41
Roasted Eggplant Salad	44
Penne with Tahini Sauce	47
Roasted Veggies	49
Zucchini Pasta	52
Asparagus Pasta	55
Feta & Spinach Pita Bake	58
DESSERT RECIPES	61
Chocolate Ganache	61
Chocolate Covered Strawberries	63
Strawberry Angel Food Dessert	65

Fruit Pizza	66
Bananas Foster	69
Cranberry Orange Cookies	71
Key Lime Pie	74
Rhubarb Strawberry Crunch	75
Chocolate Chip Banana Dessert	77
Apple Pie Filling	80
Ice Cream Sandwich Dessert	82
Cranberry and Pistachio Biscotti	84
Cream Puff Dessert	87
Fresh Peach Dessert	90
Blueberry Dessert	92
Good Sweet	94
A Taste of Dessert	94
Honey Carrots	96
Fresh Cherry Treat	97
Milky Peachy Dessert	98
Citrus Sections	99
After Meal Apples	100
Warm Nut Bites	101
Dipped Sprouts	102
Pecans and Cheese	103
Hazelnut Cookies	104
Fruit Dessert Nachos	106
Honey Yogurt with Berries	108

© Copyright 2020 by Alexangel Kitchen - All rights reserved.

The following Book is reproduced below with the goal of providing information that is as accurate and reliable as possible. Regardless, purchasing this Book can be seen as consent to the fact that both the publisher and the author of this book are in no way experts on the topics discussed within and that any recommendations or suggestions that are made herein are for entertainment purposes only. Professionals should be consulted as needed prior to undertaking any of the action endorsed herein.

This declaration is deemed fair and valid by both the American Bar Association and the Committee of Publishers Association and is legally binding throughout the United States.

Furthermore, the transmission, duplication, or reproduction of any of the following work including specific information will be considered an illegal act irrespective of if it is done electronically or in print. This extends to creating a secondary or tertiary copy of the work or a recorded copy and is only allowed with the express written consent from the Publisher. All additional right reserved.

The information in the following pages is broadly considered a truthful and accurate account of facts and as such, any inattention, use, or misuse of the information in question by the reader will render any resulting actions solely under their purview. There are no scenarios in which the publisher or the original author of this work can be in any fashion deemed liable for any hardship or damages that may befall them after undertaking information described herein.

Additionally, the information in the following pages is intended only for informational purposes and should thus be thought of as universal. As befitting its nature, it is presented without assurance regarding its prolonged validity or interim quality. Trademarks that are mentioned are done without written consent and can in no way be considered an endorsement from the trademark holder.

SALADS RECIPES

Beans and Cucumber Salad

Preparation Time: 10 minutes

Cooking Time: 0 minutes

Servings: 4

Size/ Portion: 2 cups

Ingredients:

- 15 oz. canned great northern beans
- 2 tablespoons olive oil
- ½ cup baby arugula
- 1 cup cucumber
- 1 tablespoon parsley
- 2 tomatoes, cubed
- 2 tablespoon balsamic vinegar

Directions:

1. Mix the beans with the cucumber and the rest of the ingredients in a large bowl, toss and serve cold.

Nutrition: 233 calories 9g fat 8g protein

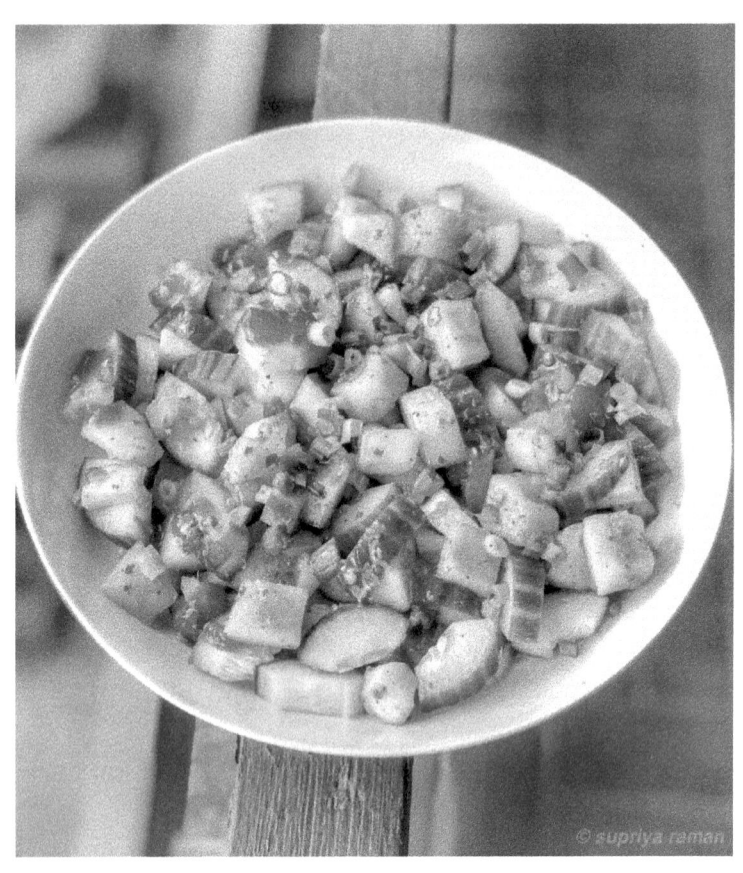

Tomato and Avocado Salad

Preparation Time: 10 minutes

Cooking Time: 0 minutes

Servings: 4

Size/ Portion: 2 cups

Ingredients:

- 1-pound cherry tomatoes
- 2 avocados
- 1 sweet onion, chopped
- 2 tablespoons lemon juice
- 1 and ½ tablespoons olive oil
- Handful basil, chopped

Directions:

1. Mix the tomatoes with the avocados and the rest of the ingredients in a serving bowl, toss and serve right away.

Nutrition: 148 Calories 7.8g Fat 5.5g Protein

Arugula Salad

Preparation Time: 5 minutes

Cooking Time: 0 minutes

Servings: 4

Size/ Portion: 2 cups

Ingredients:

- Arugula leaves (4 cups)
- Cherry tomatoes (1 cup)
- Pine nuts (.25 cup)
- Rice vinegar (1 tbsp.)
- Olive/grapeseed oil (2 tbsp.)
- Grated parmesan cheese (.25 cup)
- Black pepper & salt (as desired)
- Large sliced avocado (1)

Directions:

1. Peel and slice the avocado. Rinse and dry the arugula leaves, grate the cheese, and slice the cherry tomatoes into halves.
2. Combine the arugula, pine nuts, tomatoes, oil, vinegar, salt, pepper, and cheese.
3. Toss the salad to mix and portion it onto plates with the avocado slices to serve.

Nutrition: 257 Calories 23g Fats 6.1g Protein

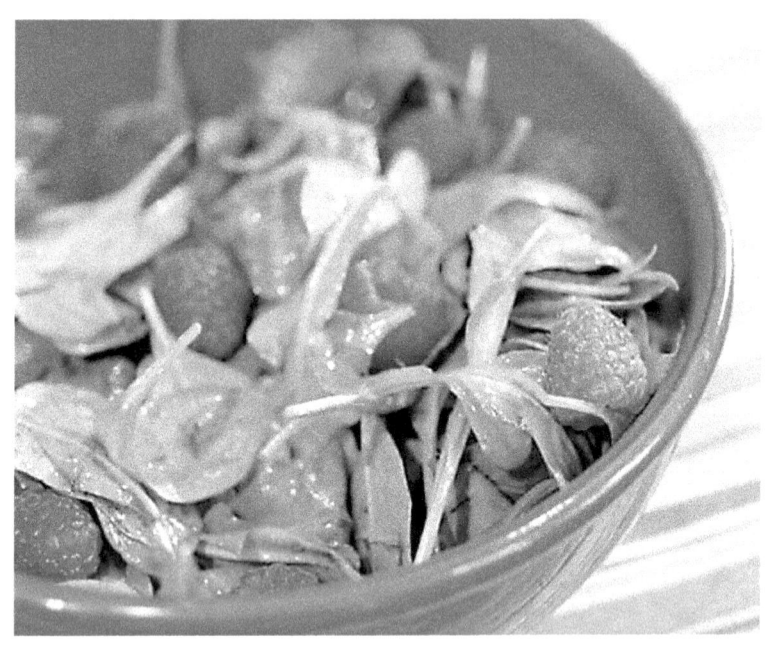

Chickpea Salad

Preparation Time: 15 minutes

Cooking Time: 0 minutes

Servings: 4

Size/ Portion: 2 cups

Ingredients:

- Cooked chickpeas (15 oz.)
- Diced Roma tomato (1)
- Diced green medium bell pepper (half of 1)
- Fresh parsley (1 tbsp.)
- Small white onion (1)
- Minced garlic (.5 tsp.)
- Lemon (1 juiced)

Directions:

1. Chop the tomato, green pepper, and onion. Mince the garlic. Combine each of the fixings into a salad bowl and toss well.
2. Cover the salad to chill for at least 15 minutes in the fridge. Serve when ready.

Nutrition: 163 Calories 7g Fats 4g Protein

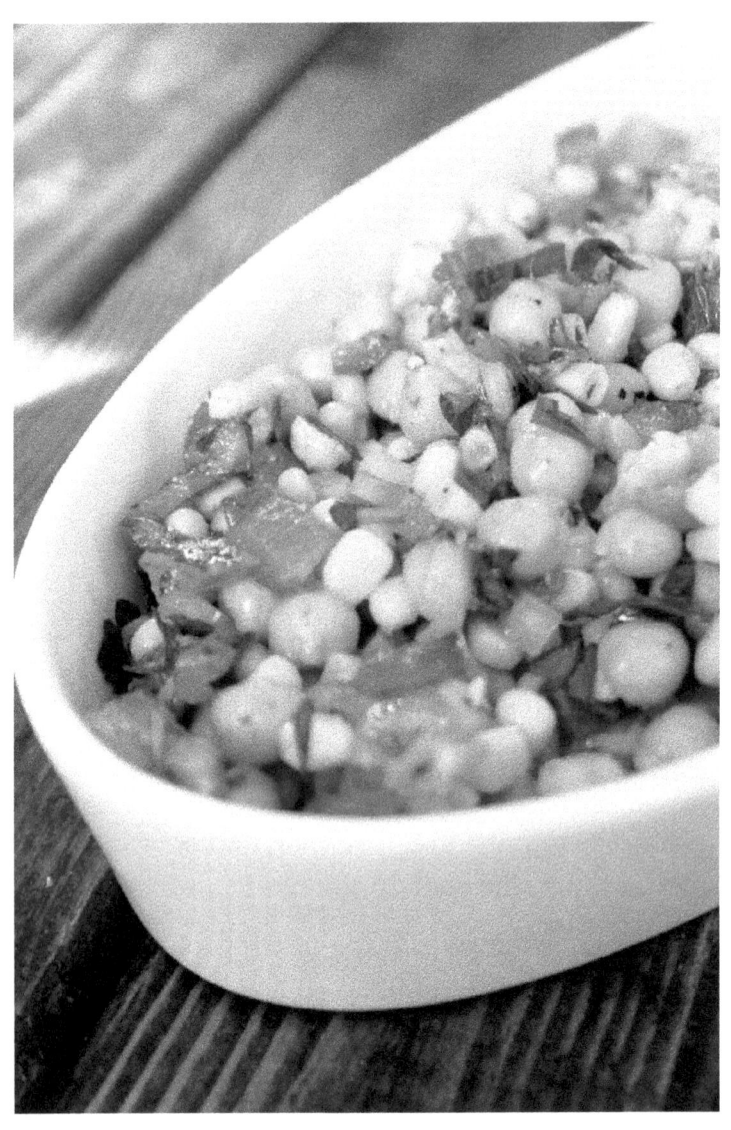

Chopped Israeli Mediterranean Pasta Salad

Preparation Time: 15 minutes

Cooking Time: 2 minutes

Servings: 8

Size/ Portion: 2 cups

Ingredients:

- Small bow tie or other small pasta (.5 lb.)
- 1/3 cup Cucumber
- 1/3 cup Radish
- 1/3 cup Tomato
- 1/3 cup Yellow bell pepper
- 1/3 cup Orange bell pepper
- 1/3 cup Black olives
- 1/3 cup Green olives
- 1/3 cup Red onions
- 1/3 cup Pepperoncini
- 1/3 cup Feta cheese
- 1/3 cup Fresh thyme leaves
- Dried oregano (1 tsp.)

Dressing:

- 0.25 cup + more, olive oil
- juice of 1 lemon

Directions:

1. Slice the green olives into halves. Dice the feta and pepperoncini. Finely dice the remainder of the veggies.

2. Prepare a pot of water with the salt, and simmer the pasta until its al dente (checking at two minutes under the listed time). Rinse and drain in cold water.

3. Combine a small amount of oil with the pasta. Add the salt, pepper, oregano, thyme, and veggies. Pour in the rest of the oil, lemon juice, and mix and fold in the grated feta.

4. Pop it into the fridge within two hours, best if overnight. Taste test and adjust the seasonings to your liking; add fresh thyme.

Nutrition: 65 Calories 5.6g Fats 0.8g Protein

Feta Tomato Salad

Preparation Time: 5 minutes

Cooking Time: 0 minutes

Servings: 4

Size/ Portion: 2 cups

Ingredients:

- Balsamic vinegar (2 tbsp.)
- Freshly minced basil (1.5 tsp.) or dried (.5 tsp.)
- Salt (.5 tsp.)
- Coarsely chopped sweet onion (.5 cup)
- Olive oil (2 tbsp.)
- Cherry or grape tomatoes (1 lb.)
- Crumbled feta cheese (.25 cup.)

Directions:

1. Whisk the salt, basil, and vinegar. Toss the onion into the vinegar mixture for 5 minutes
2. Slice the tomatoes into halves and stir in the tomatoes, feta cheese, and oil to serve.

Nutrition: 121 Calories 9g Fats 3g Protein

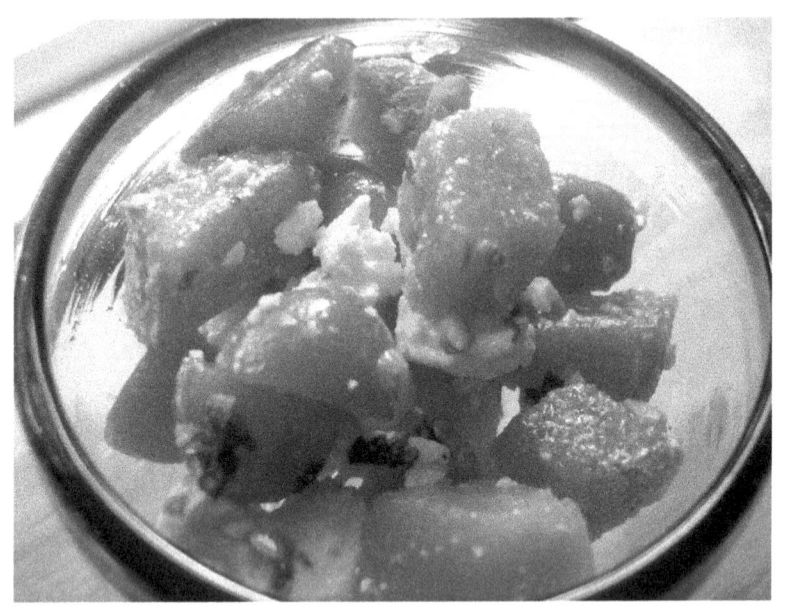

Greek Pasta Salad

Preparation Time: 5 minutes

Cooking Time: 11 minutes

Servings: 4

Size/ Portion: 2 cups

Ingredients:

- Penne pasta (1 cup)
- Lemon juice (1.5 tsp.)
- Red wine vinegar (2 tbsp.)
- Garlic (1 clove)
- Dried oregano (1 tsp.)
- Black pepper and sea salt (as desired)
- Olive oil (.33 cup)
- Halved cherry tomatoes (5)
- Red onion (half of 1 small)
- Green & red bell pepper (half of 1 - each)
- Cucumber (¼ of 1)
- Black olives (.25 cup)
- Crumbled feta cheese (.25 cup)

Directions:

1. Slice the cucumber and olives. Chop/dice the onion, peppers, and garlic. Slice the tomatoes into halves.

2. Arrange a large pot with water and salt using the high-temperature setting. Once it's boiling, add the pasta and cook for 11 minutes Rinse it using cold water and drain in a colander.

3. Whisk the oil, juice, salt, pepper, vinegar, oregano, and garlic. Combine the cucumber, cheese, olives, peppers, pasta, onions, and tomatoes in a large salad dish.

4. Add the vinaigrette over the pasta and toss. Chill in the fridge (covered) for about three hours and serve as desired.

Nutrition: 307 Calories 23.6g Fat 5.4g Protein

Watermelon Salad

Preparation Time: 18 minutes

Cooking Time: 0 minute

Serving: 6

Size/ Portion: 2 cups

Ingredients:

- ¼ teaspoon sea salt
- ¼ teaspoon black pepper
- 1 tablespoon balsamic vinegar
- 1 cantaloupe, quartered & seeded
- 12 watermelon, small & seedless
- 2 cups mozzarella balls, fresh
- 1/3 cup basil, fresh & torn
- 2 tablespoons olive oil

Directions:

1. Scoop out balls of cantaloupe, and the put them in a colander over bowl.
2. With a melon baller slice the watermelon.
3. Allow your fruit to drain for ten minutes, and then refrigerate the juice.
4. Wipe the bowl dry, and then place your fruit in it.

5. Stir in basil, oil, vinegar, mozzarella and tomatoes before seasoning.

6. Mix well and serve.

Nutrition: 218 Calories 10g Protein 13g Fat

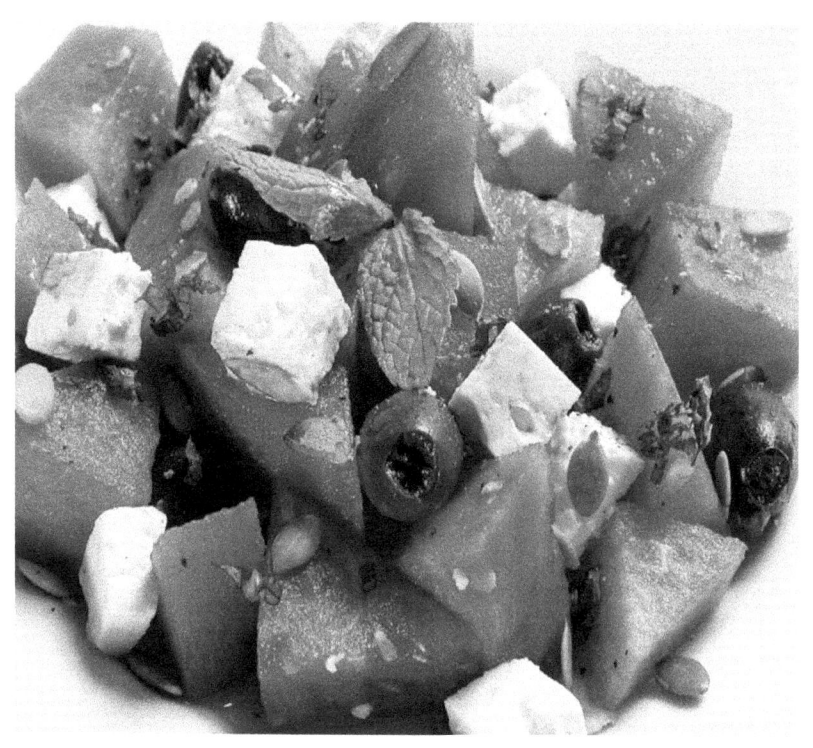

Orange Celery Salad

Preparation Time: 16 minutes

Cooking Time: 0 minute

Serving: 6

Size/ Portion: 2 cups

Ingredients:

- 1 tablespoon lemon juice, fresh
- ¼ teaspoon sea salt, fine
- ¼ teaspoon black pepper
- 1 tablespoon olive brine
- 1 tablespoon olive oil
- ¼ cup red onion, sliced
- ½ cup green olives
- 2 oranges, peeled & sliced
- 3 celery stalks, sliced diagonally in ½ inch slices

Directions:

1. Put your oranges, olives, onion and celery in a shallow bowl.
2. Stir oil, olive brine and lemon juice, pour this over your salad.
3. Season with salt and pepper before serving.

Nutrition: 65 Calories 2g Protein 0.2g Fat

Roasted Broccoli Salad

Preparation Time: 9 minutes

Cooking Time: 17 minutes

Serving: 4

Size/ portion: 2 cups

Ingredients:

- 1 lb. broccoli
- 3 tablespoons olive oil, divided
- 1-pint cherry tomatoes
- 1 ½ teaspoons honey
- 3 cups cubed bread, whole grain
- 1 tablespoon balsamic vinegar
- ½ teaspoon black pepper
- ¼ teaspoon sea salt, fine
- grated parmesan for serving

Directions:

1. Set oven to 450, and then place rimmed baking sheet.
2. Drizzle your broccoli with a tablespoon of oil, and toss to coat.
3. Take out from oven, and spoon the broccoli. Leave oil at bottom of the bowl and add in your tomatoes, toss

to coat, then mix tomatoes with a tablespoon of honey. Place on the same baking sheet.

4. Roast for fifteen minutes, and stir halfway through your cooking time.

5. Add in your bread, and then roast for three more minutes.

6. Whisk two tablespoons of oil, vinegar, and remaining honey. Season. Pour this over your broccoli mix to serve.

Nutrition: 226 Calories 7g Protein 12g Fat

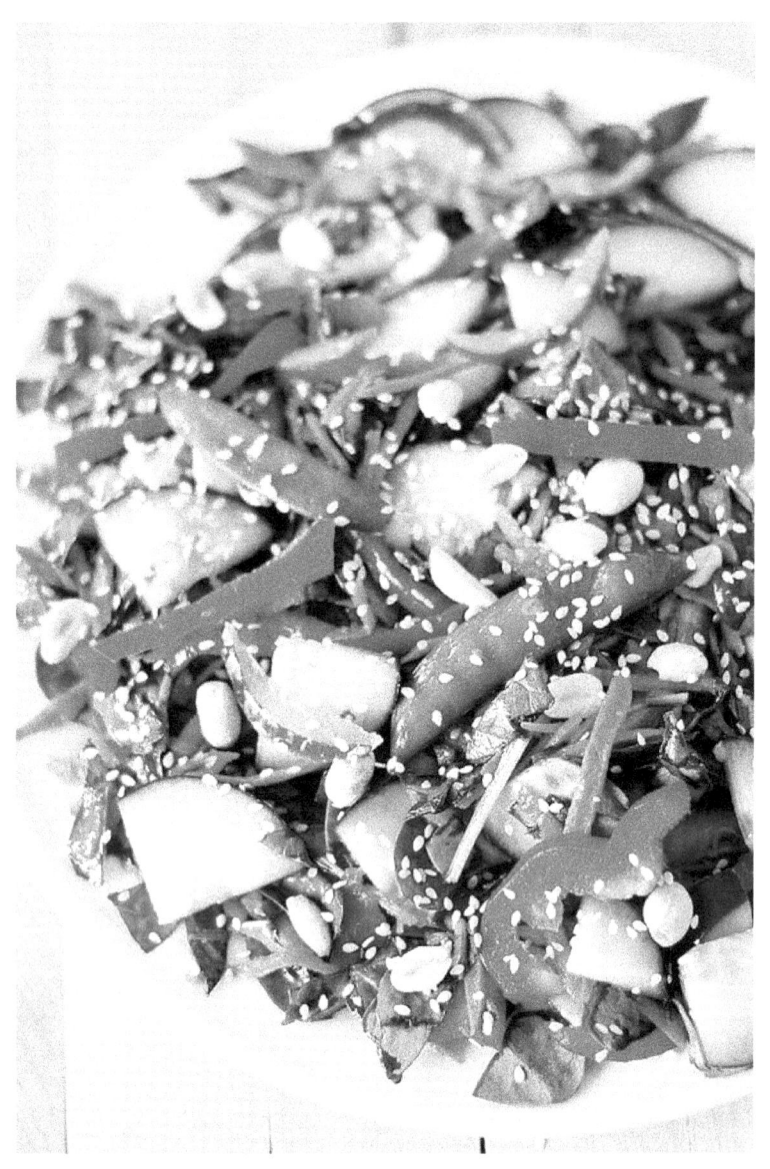

Tomato Salad

Preparation Time: 22 minutes

Cooking Time: 0 minute

Serving: 4

Size/ portion: 2 cups

Ingredients:

- 1 cucumber, sliced
- ¼ cup sun dried tomatoes, chopped
- 1 lb. tomatoes, cubed
- ½ cup black olives
- 1 red onion, sliced
- 1 tablespoon balsamic vinegar
- ¼ cup parsley, fresh & chopped
- 2 tablespoons olive oil

Directions:

1. Get out a bowl and combine all of your vegetables together. To make your dressing mix all your seasoning, olive oil and vinegar.
2. Toss with your salad and serve fresh.

Nutrition: 126 Calories 2.1g Protein 9.2g Fat

Feta Beet Salad

Preparation Time: 16 minutes

Cooking Time: 0 minute

Serving: 4

Size/ Portion: 2 cups

Ingredients:

- 6 Red Beets, Cooked & Peeled
- 3 Ounces Feta Cheese, Cubed
- 2 Tablespoons Olive Oil
- 2 Tablespoons Balsamic Vinegar

Directions:

1. Combine everything together, and then serve.

Nutrition: 230 Calories 7.3g Protein 12g Fat

Cauliflower & Tomato Salad

Preparation Time: 17 minutes

Cooking Time: 0 minute

Serving: 4

Size/ Portion: 2 cups

Ingredients:

- 1 Head Cauliflower, Chopped
- 2 Tablespoons Parsley, Fresh & chopped

- 2 Cups Cherry Tomatoes, Halved
- 2 Tablespoons Lemon Juice, Fresh
- 2 Tablespoons Pine Nuts

Directions:

1. Incorporate lemon juice, cherry tomatoes, cauliflower and parsley and season well. Sprinkle the pine nuts, and mix.

Nutrition: 64 Calories 2.8g Protein 3.3g Fat

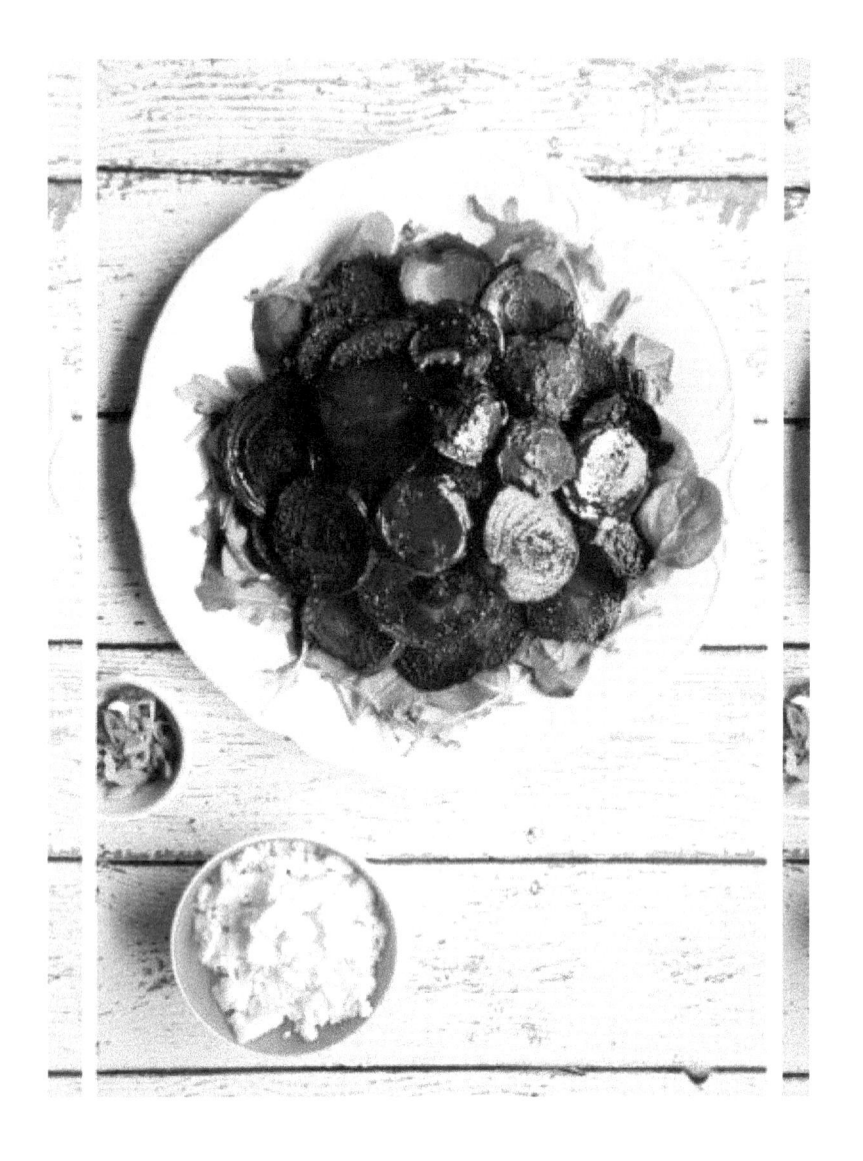

Tahini Spinach

Preparation Time: 11 minutes

Cooking Time: 6 minutes

Serving: 3

Size/ Portion: 2 cups

Ingredients:

- 10 spinach, chopped
- ½ cup water
- 1 tablespoon tahini
- 2 cloves garlic, minced
- ¼ teaspoon cumin
- ¼ teaspoon paprika
- ¼ teaspoon cayenne pepper
- 1/3 cup red wine vinegar

Direction:

1. Add your spinach and water to the saucepan, and then boil it on high heat. Once boiling reduce to low, and cover. Allow it to cook on simmer for five minutes.

2. Add in your garlic, cumin, cayenne, red wine vinegar, paprika and tahini. Whisk well, and season with salt and pepper.

3. Drain your spinach and top with tahini sauce to serve.

Nutrition: 69 Calories 5g Protein 3g Fat

Pilaf with Cream Cheese

Preparation Time: 11 minutes

Cooking Time: 34 minutes

Serving: 6

Size/ Portion: 2 cups

Ingredients:

- 2 cups yellow long grain rice, parboiled
- 1 cup onion
- 4 green onions
- 3 tablespoons butter
- 3 tablespoons vegetable broth
- 2 teaspoons cayenne pepper
- 1 teaspoon paprika
- ½ teaspoon cloves, minced
- 2 tablespoons mint leaves
- 1 bunch fresh mint leaves to garnish
- 1 tablespoons olive oil

Cheese Cream:

- 3 tablespoons olive oil
- sea salt & black pepper to taste
- 9 ounces cream cheese

Directions:

1. Start by heating your oven to 360, and then get out a pan. Heat your butter and olive oil together, and cook your onions and spring onions for two minutes.

2. Add in your salt, pepper, paprika, cloves, vegetable broth, rice and remaining seasoning. S

3. Sauté for three minutes.

4. Wrap with foil, and bake for another half hour. Allow it to cool.

5. Mix in the cream cheese, cheese, olive oil, salt and pepper. Serve your pilaf garnished with fresh mint leaves.

Nutrition: 364 Calories 5g Protein 30g Fat

Easy Spaghetti Squash

Preparation Time: 13 minutes

Cooking Time: 45 minutes

Serving: 6

Size/ Portion: 2 ounces

Ingredients:

- 2 spring onions, chopped fine
- 3 cloves garlic, minced
- 1 zucchini, diced
- 1 red bell pepper, diced
- 1 tablespoon Italian seasoning
- 1 tomato, small & chopped fine
- 1 tablespoons parsley, fresh & chopped
- pinch lemon pepper
- dash sea salt, fine
- 4 ounces feta cheese, crumbled
- 3 Italian sausage links, casing removed
- 2 tablespoons olive oil
- 1 spaghetti sauce, halved lengthwise

Directions:

1. Prep oven to 350, and get out a large baking sheet. Coat it with cooking spray, and then put your squash on it with the cut side down.

2. Bake at 350 for forty-five minutes. It should be tender.

3. Turn the squash over, and bake for five more minutes. Scrape the strands into a larger bowl.

4. Cook tablespoon of olive oil in a skillet, and then add in your Italian sausage. Cook at eight minutes before removing it and placing it in a bowl.

5. Add another tablespoon of olive oil to the skillet and cook your garlic and onions until softened. This will take five minutes. Throw in your Italian seasoning, red peppers and zucchini. Cook for another five minutes. Your vegetables should be softened.

6. Mix in your feta cheese and squash, cooking until the cheese has melted.

7. Stir in your sausage, and then season with lemon pepper and salt. Serve with parsley and tomato.

Nutrition: 423 Calories 18g Protein 30g Fat

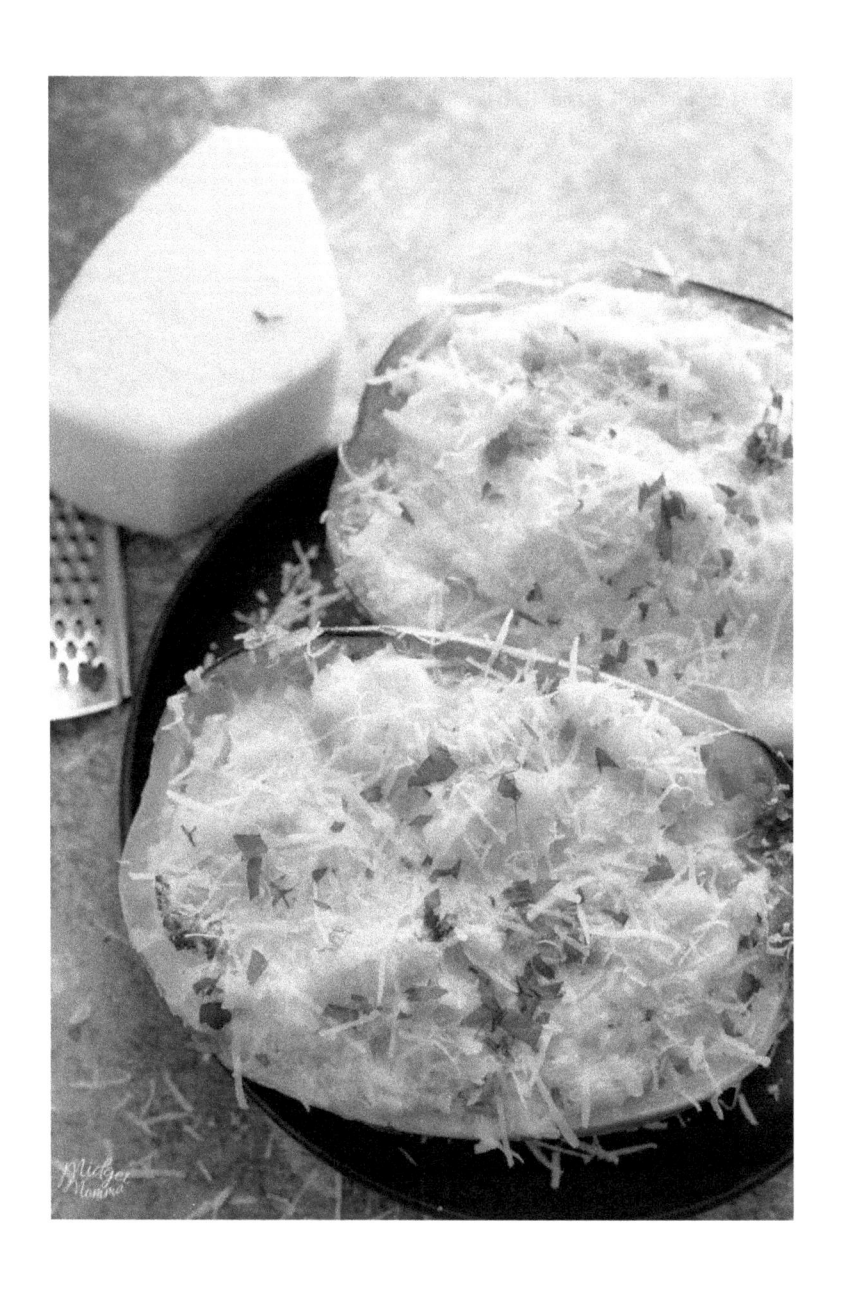

Roasted Eggplant Salad

Preparation Time: 14 minutes

Cooking Time: 36 minutes

Serving: 6

Size/ Portion: 2 cups

Ingredients:

- 1 red onion, sliced
- 2 tablespoons parsley
- 1 teaspoon thyme
- 2 cups cherry tomatoes
- 1 teaspoon oregano
- 3 tablespoons olive oil
- 1 teaspoon basil
- 3 eggplants, peeled & cubed

Directions:

1. Start by heating your oven to 350.
2. Season your eggplant with basil, salt, pepper, oregano, thyme and olive oil.
3. Arrange it on a baking tray, and bake for a half hour.
4. Toss with your remaining ingredients before serving.

Nutrition: 148 Calories 3.5g Protein 7.7g Fat

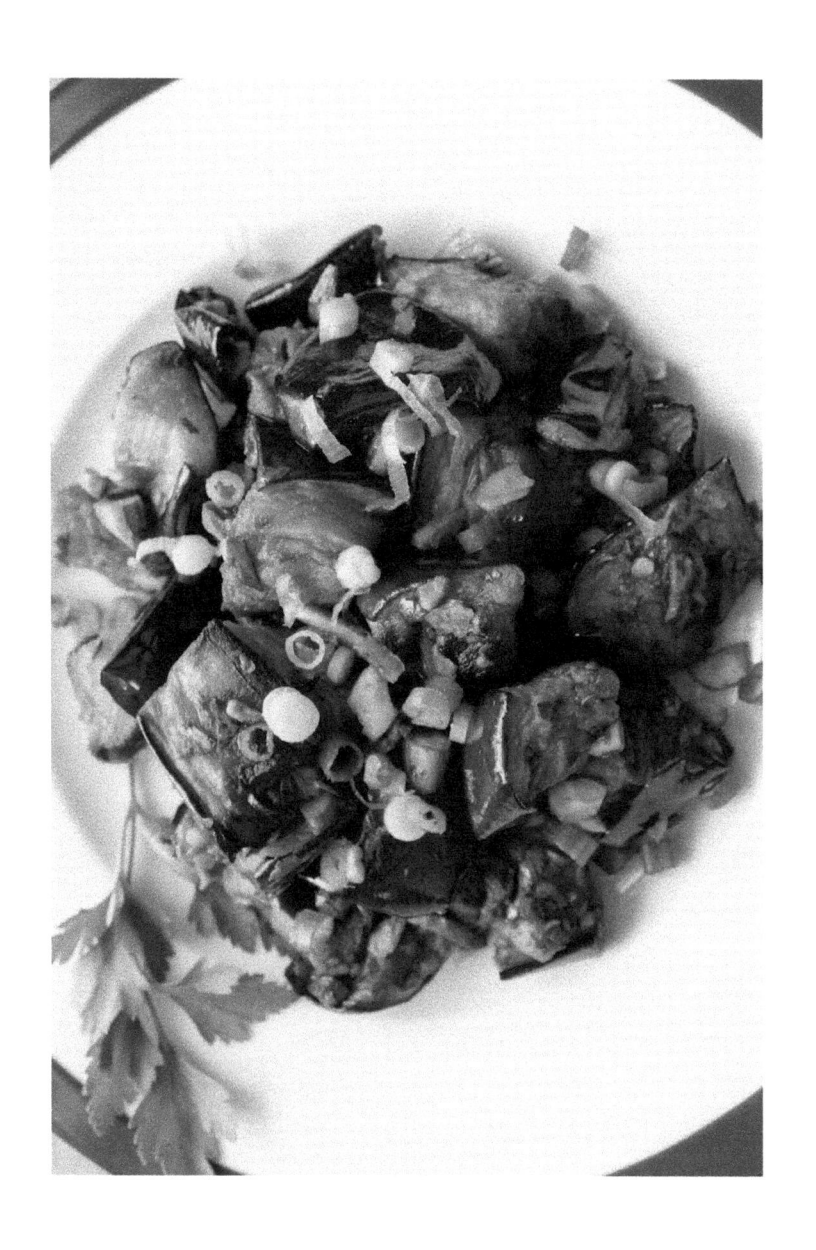

Penne with Tahini Sauce

Preparation Time: 16 minutes

Cooking Time: 22 minutes

Serving: 8

Size/ Portion: 2 ounces

Ingredients:

- 1/3 cup water
- 1 cup yogurt, plain
- 1/8 cup lemon juice
- 3 tablespoons tahini
- 3 cloves garlic
- 1 onion, chopped
- ¼ cup olive oil
- 2 portobello mushrooms, large & sliced
- ½ red bell pepper, diced
- 16 ounces penne pasta
- ½ cup parsley, fresh & chopped

Directions:

1. Start by getting out a pot and bring a pot of salted water to a boil. Cook your pasta al dente per package instructions.

2. Mix your lemon juice and tahini together, and then place it in a food processor. Process with garlic, water and yogurt.

3. Situate pan over medium heat. Heat up your oil, and cook your onions until soft.

4. Add in your mushroom and continue to cook until softened.

5. Add in your bell pepper, and cook until crispy.

6. Drain your pasta, and then toss with your tahini sauce, top with parsley and pepper and serve with vegetables.

Nutrition: 332 Calories 11g Proteins 12g Fat

Roasted Veggies

Preparation Time: 14 minutes

Cooking Time: 26 minutes

Serving: 12

Size/ Portion: 2 cups

Ingredients:

- 6 cloves garlic
- 6 tablespoons olive oil
- 1 fennel bulb, diced
- 1 zucchini, diced
- 2 red bell peppers, diced
- 6 potatoes, large & diced
- 2 teaspoons sea salt
- ½ cup balsamic vinegar
- ¼ cup rosemary, chopped & fresh
- 2 teaspoons vegetable bouillon powder

Directions:

1. Start by heating your oven to 400.
2. Get out a baking dish and place your potatoes, fennel, zucchini, garlic and fennel on a baking dish, drizzling with olive oil. Sprinkle with salt, bouillon powder, and rosemary. Mix well, and then bake at 450 for

thirty to forty minutes. Mix your vinegar into the vegetables before serving.

Nutrition: 675 Calories 13g Protein 21g Fat

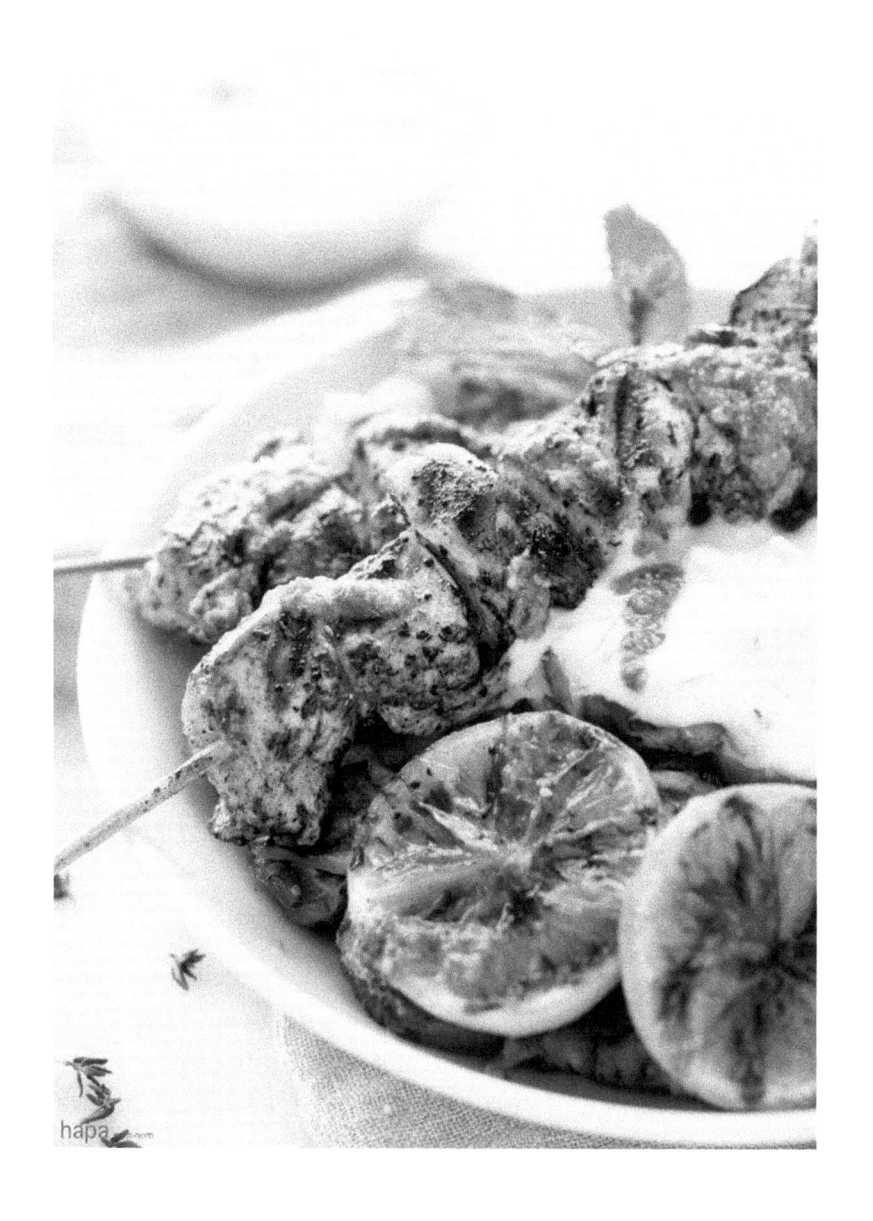

Zucchini Pasta

Preparation Time: 9 minutes

Cooking Time: 32 minutes

Serving: 4

Size/ Portion: 2 ounces

Ingredients:

- 3 tablespoons olive oil
- 2 cloves garlic, minced
- 3 zucchinis, large & diced
- sea salt & black pepper to taste
- ½ cup milk, 2%
- ¼ teaspoon nutmeg
- 1 tablespoon lemon juice, fresh
- ½ cup parmesan, grated
- 8 ounces uncooked farfalle pasta

Directions:

1. Get out a skillet and place it over medium heat, and then heat up the oil. Add in your garlic and cook for a minute. Stir often so that it doesn't burn. Add in your salt, pepper and zucchini. Stir well, and cook covered for fifteen minutes. During this time, you'll want to stir the mixture twice.

2. Get out a microwave safe bowl, and heat the milk for thirty seconds. Stir in your nutmeg, and then pour it into the skillet. Cook uncovered for five minutes. Stir occasionally to keep from burning.

3. Get out a stockpot and cook your pasta per package instructions. Drain the pasta, and then save two tablespoons of pasta water.

4. Stir everything together, and add in the cheese and lemon juice and pasta water.

Nutrition: 410 Calories 15g Protein 17g Fat

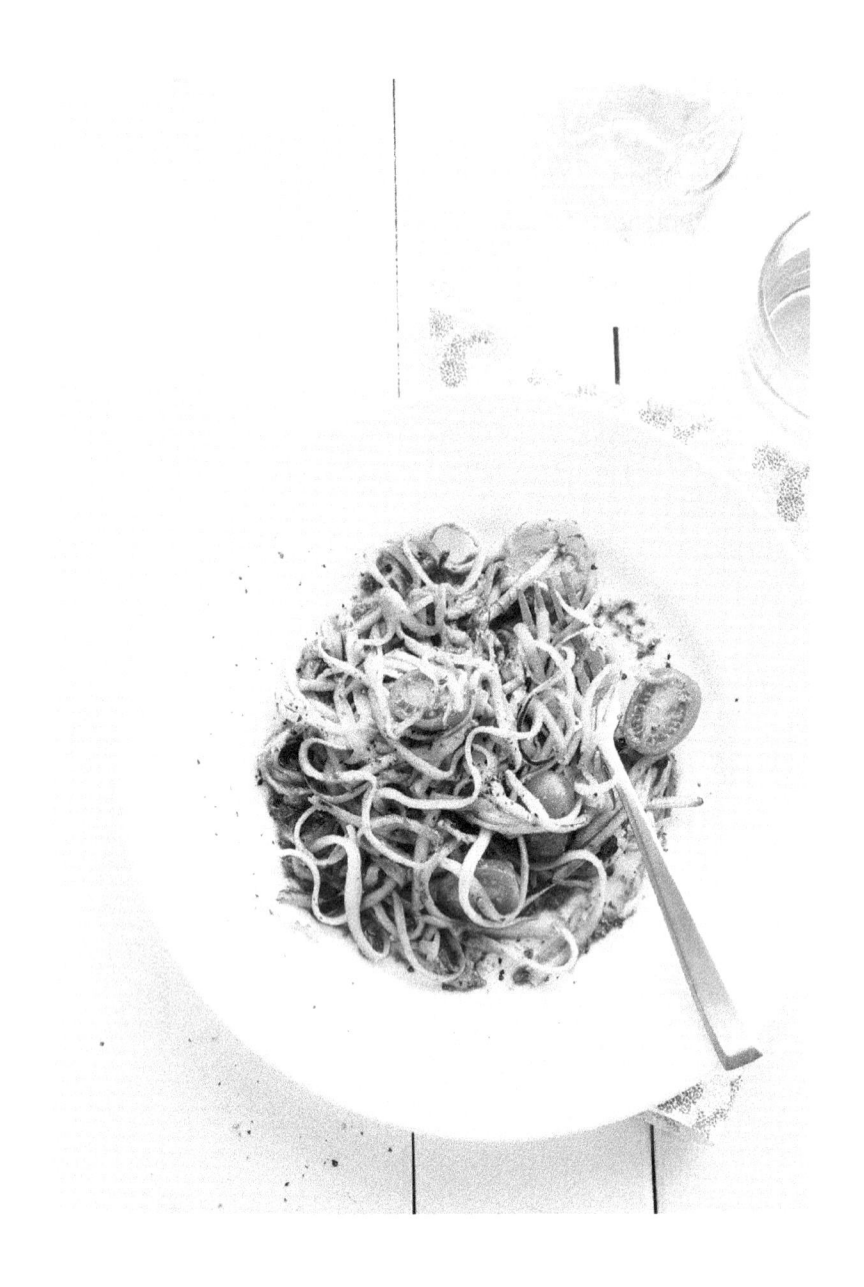

Asparagus Pasta

Preparation Time: 8 minutes

Cooking Time: 33 minutes

Serving: 6

Size/ Portion: 2 ounces

Ingredients:

- 8 ounces farfalle pasta, uncooked
- 1 ½ cups asparagus
- 1-pint grape tomatoes, halved
- 2 tablespoons olive oil
- 2 cups mozzarella, fresh & drained
- 1/3 cup basil leaves, fresh & torn
- 2 tablespoons balsamic vinegar

Directions:

1. Start by heating the oven to 400, and then get out a stockpot. Cook your pasta per package instructions, and reserve ¼ cup of pasta water.
2. Get out a bowl and toss the tomatoes, oil, asparagus, and season with salt and pepper. Spread this mixture on a baking sheet, and bake for fifteen minutes. Stir twice in this time.
3. Remove your vegetables from the oven, and then add the cooked pasta to your baking sheet. Mix with a few

tablespoons of pasta water so that your sauce becomes smoother.

4. Mix in your basil and mozzarella, drizzling with balsamic vinegar. Serve warm.

Nutrition: 307 Calories 18g Protein 14g Fat

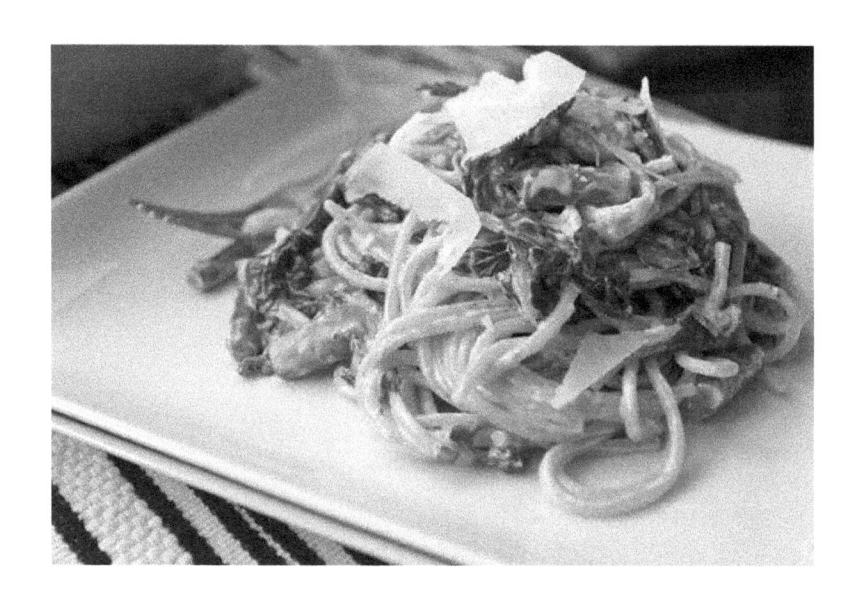

Feta & Spinach Pita Bake

Preparation Time: 11 minutes

Cooking Time: 36 minutes

Serving: 6

Size/ Portion: 2 ounces

Ingredients:

- 2 roma tomatoes
- 6 whole wheat pita bread
- 1 jar sun dried tomato pesto
- 4 mushrooms, fresh & sliced
- 1 bunch spinach
- 2 tablespoons parmesan cheese
- 3 tablespoons olive oil
- ½ cup feta cheese

Directions:

1. Start by heating the oven to 350, and get to your pita bread. Spread the tomato pesto on the side of each one. Put them in a baking pan with the tomato side up.

2. Top with tomatoes, spinach, mushrooms, parmesan and feta. Drizzle with olive oil and season with pepper.

3. Bake for twelve minutes, and then serve cut into quarters.

Nutrition: 350 Calories 12g Protein 17g Fat

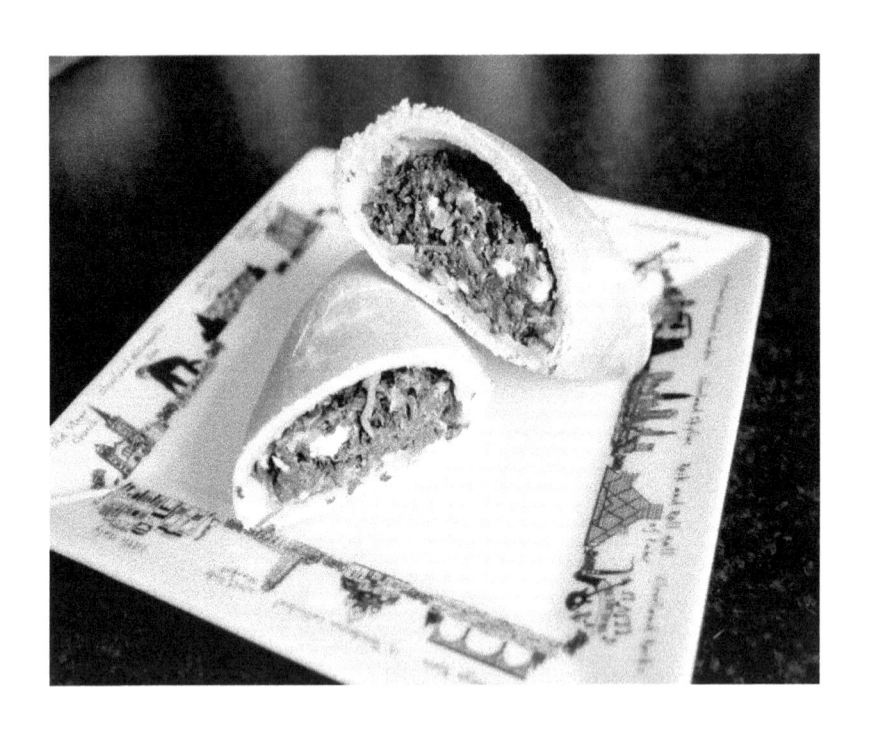

DESSERT RECIPES

Chocolate Ganache

Preparation Time: 10 minutes

Cooking Time: 16 minutes

Servings: 16

Size/ Portion: 2 tablespoons

Ingredients

- 9 ounces bittersweet chocolate, chopped
- 1 cup heavy cream
- 1 tablespoon dark rum (optional)

Direction

1. Situate chocolate in a medium bowl. Cook cream in a small saucepan over medium heat.
2. Bring to a boil. When the cream has reached a boiling point, pour the chopped chocolate over it and beat until smooth. Stir the rum if desired.
3. Allow the ganache to cool slightly before you pour it on a cake. Begin in the middle of the cake and work outside. For a fluffy icing or chocolate filling, let it cool until thick and beat with a whisk until light and fluffy.

Nutrition: 142 calories 10.8g fat 1.4g protein

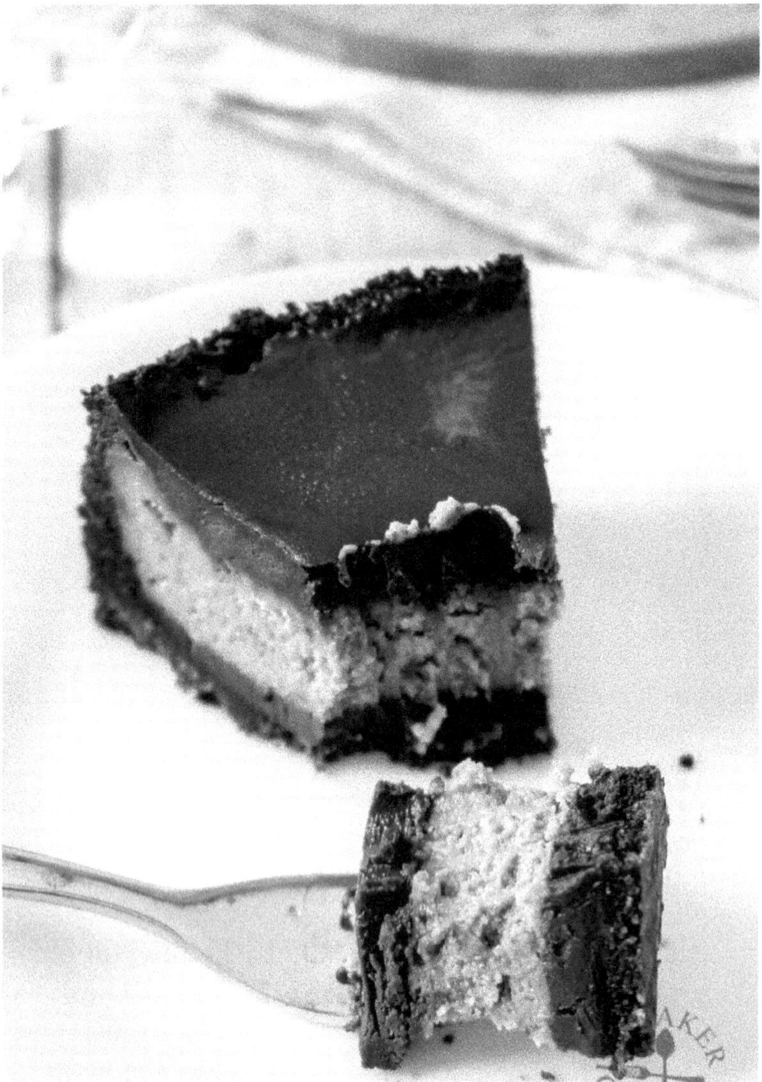

Chocolate Covered Strawberries

Preparation Time: 15 minutes

Cooking Time: 0 minute

Servings: 24

Size/ Portion: 2 pieces

Ingredients

- 16 ounces milk chocolate chips
- 2 tablespoons shortening
- 1-pound fresh strawberries with leaves

Direction

1. In a bain-marie, melt chocolate and shortening, occasionally stirring until smooth. Pierce the tops of the strawberries with toothpicks and immerse them in the chocolate mixture.
2. Turn the strawberries and put the toothpick in Styrofoam so that the chocolate cools.

Nutrition: 115 calories 7.3g fat 1.4g protein

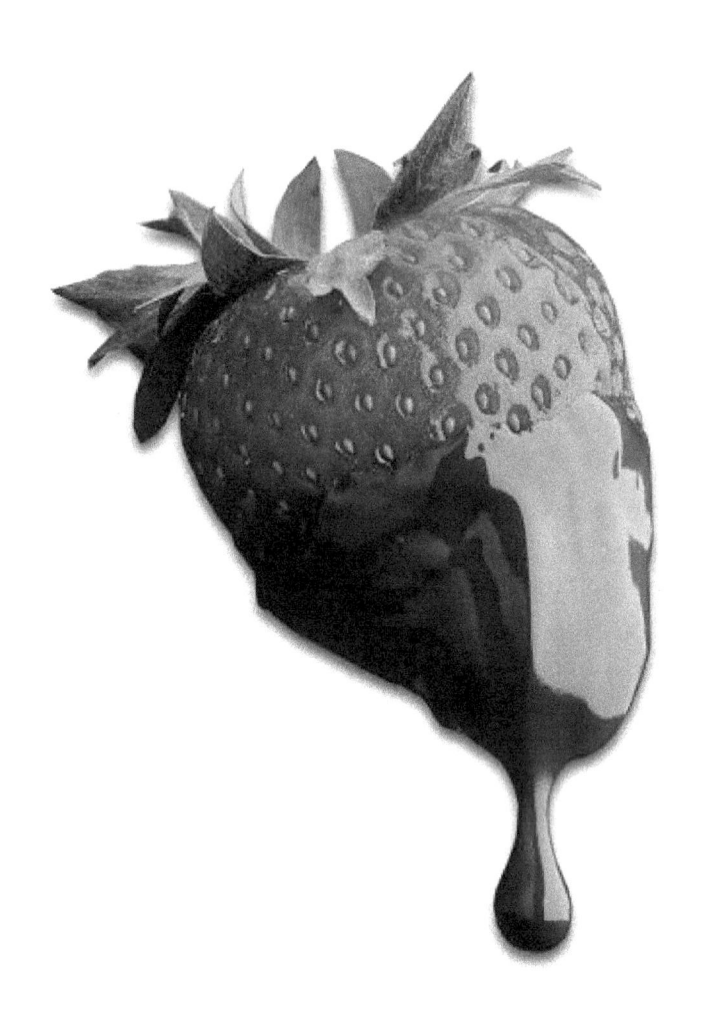

Strawberry Angel Food Dessert

Preparation Time: 15 minutes

Cooking Time: 0 minutes

Servings: 18

Size/ Portion: 1 cup

Ingredients

- 1 angel cake (10 inches)
- 2 packages of softened cream cheese
- 1 cup of white sugar
- 1 container (8 oz.) of frozen fluff, thawed
- 1 liter of fresh strawberries, sliced
- 1 jar of strawberry icing

Direction

1. Crumble the cake in a 9 x 13-inch dish.
2. Beat the cream cheese and sugar in a medium bowl until the mixture is light and fluffy. Stir in the whipped topping. Crush the cake with your hands, and spread the cream cheese mixture over the cake.
3. Combine the strawberries and the frosting in a bowl until the strawberries are well covered. Spread over the layer of cream cheese. Cool until ready to serve.

Nutrition: 261 calories 11g fat 3.2g protein

Fruit Pizza

Preparation Time: 30 minutes

Cooking Time: 0 minute

Servings: 8

Size/ Portion: 1 slice

Ingredients

- 1 (18-oz) package sugar cookie dough
- 1 (8-oz) package cream cheese, softened
- 1 (8-oz) frozen filling, defrosted
- 2 cups of freshly cut strawberries
- 1/2 cup of white sugar
- 1 pinch of salt
- 1 tablespoon corn flour
- 2 tablespoons lemon juice
- 1/2 cup orange juice
- 1/4 cup water
- 1/2 teaspoon orange zest

Direction

1. Ready oven to 175 ° C Slice the cookie dough then place it on a greased pizza pan. Press the dough flat into the mold. Bake for 10 to 12 minutes. Let cool.

2. Soften the cream cheese in a large bowl and then stir in the whipped topping. Spread over the cooled crust.

3. Start with strawberries cut in half. Situate in a circle around the outer edge. Continue with the fruit of your choice by going to the center. If you use bananas, immerse them in lemon juice. Then make a sauce with a spoon on the fruit.

4. Combine sugar, salt, corn flour, orange juice, lemon juice, and water in a pan. Boil and stir over medium heat. Boil for 1 or 2 minutes until thick. Remove from heat and add the grated orange zest. Place on the fruit.

5. Allow to cool for two hours, cut into quarters, and serve.

Nutrition: 535 calories 30g fat 5.5g protein

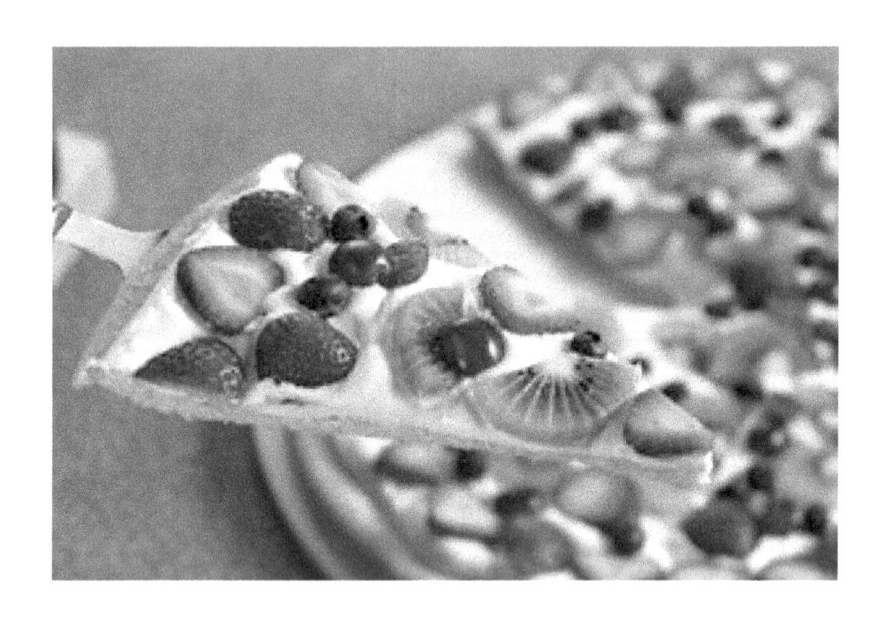

Bananas Foster

Preparation Time: 5 minutes

Cooking Time: 6 minutes

Servings: 4

Size/ Portion: 1 cup

Ingredients

- 2/3 cup dark brown sugar
- 1/4 cup butter
- 3 1/2 tablespoons rum
- 1 1/2 teaspoons vanilla extract
- 1/2 teaspoon of ground cinnamon
- 3 bananas, peeled and cut lengthwise and broad
- 1/4 cup coarsely chopped nuts
- vanilla ice cream

Direction

1. Melt the butter in a deep-frying pan over medium heat. Stir in sugar, rum, vanilla, and cinnamon.
2. When the mixture starts to bubble, place the bananas and nuts in the pan. Bake until the bananas are hot, 1 to 2 minutes. Serve immediately with vanilla ice cream.

Nutrition: 534 calories 23.8g fat 4.6g protein

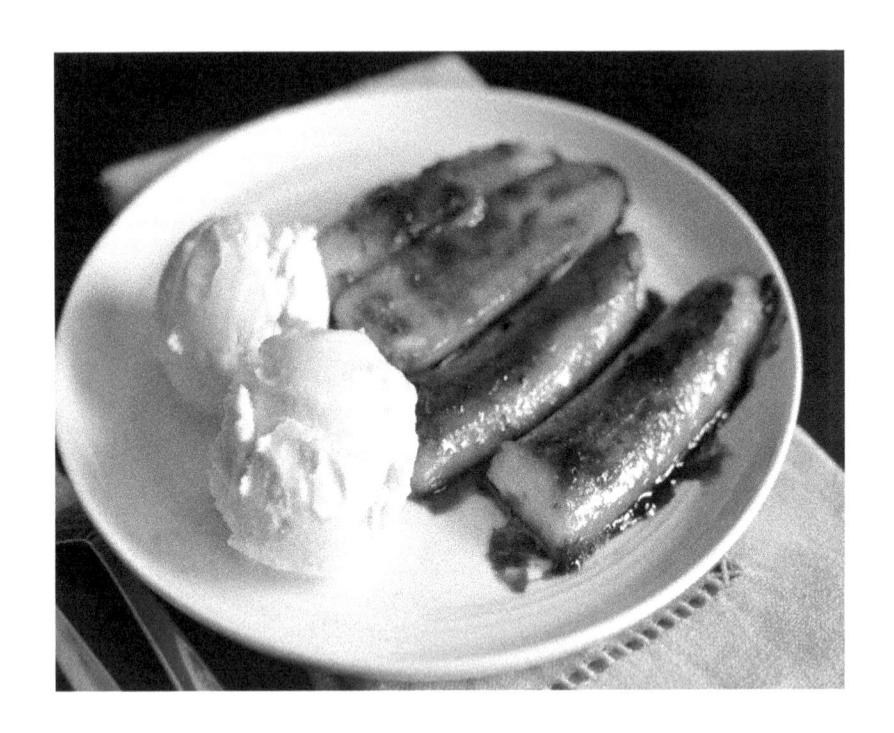

Cranberry Orange Cookies

Preparation Time: 20 minutes

Cooking Time: 16 minutes

Servings: 24

Size/ Portion: 2 cookies

Ingredients

- 1 cup of soft butter
- 1 cup of white sugar
- 1/2 cup brown sugar
- 1 egg
- 1 teaspoon grated orange peel
- 2 tablespoons orange juice
- 2 1/2 cups flour
- 1/2 teaspoon baking powder
- 1/2 teaspoon salt
- 2 cups chopped cranberries
- 1/2 cup chopped walnuts (optional)

Icing:

- 1/2 teaspoon grated orange peel
- 3 tablespoons orange juice
- 1 ½ cup confectioner's sugar

Direction

1. Preheat the oven to 190 ° C.

2. Blend butter, white sugar, and brown sugar. Beat the egg until everything is well mixed. Mix 1 teaspoon of orange zest and 2 tablespoons of orange juice. Mix the flour, baking powder, and salt; stir in the orange mixture.

3. Mix the cranberries and, if used, the nuts until well distributed. Place the dough with a spoon on ungreased baking trays.

4. Bake in the preheated oven for 12 to 14 minutes. Cool on racks.

5. In a small bowl, mix icing ingredients. Spread over cooled cookies.

Nutrition: 110 calories 4.8g fat 1.1 g protein

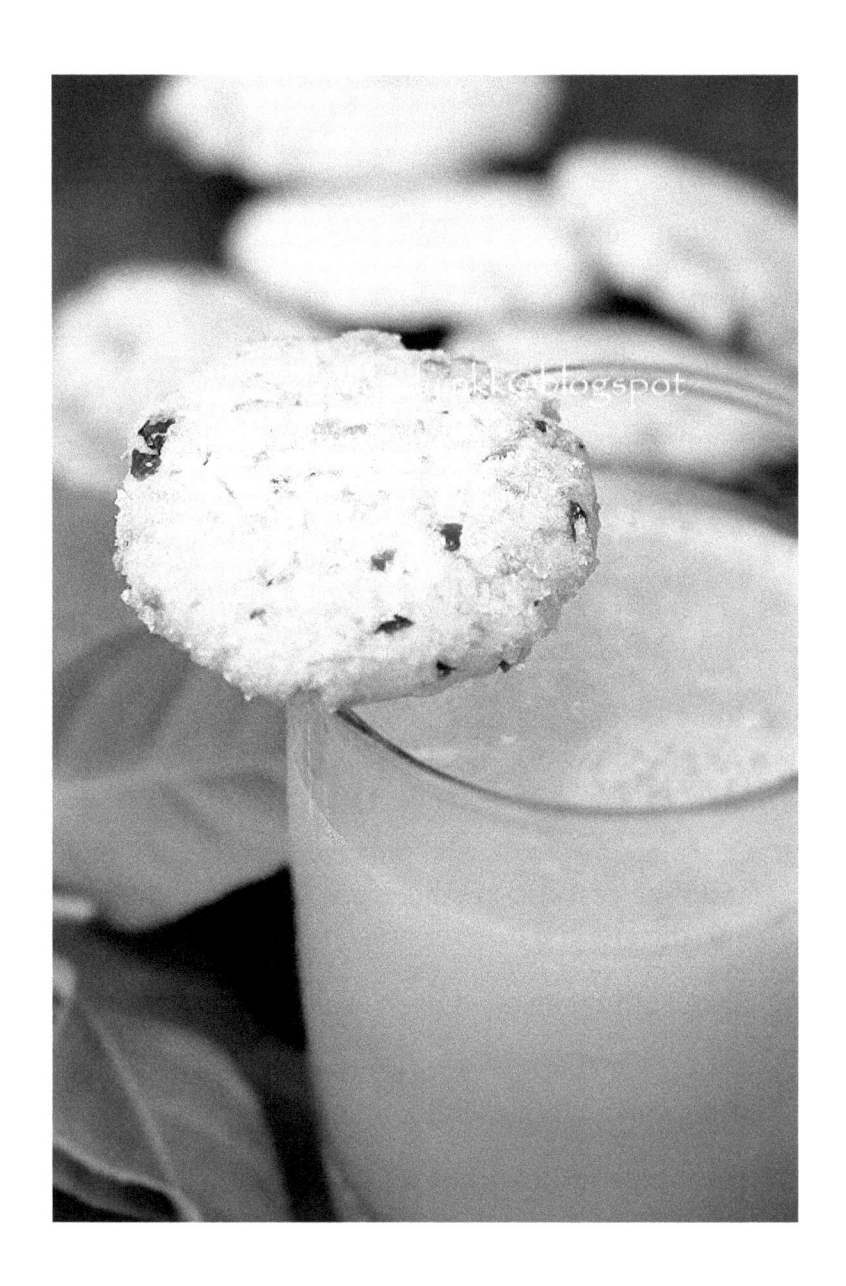

Key Lime Pie

Preparation Time: 15 minutes

Cooking Time: 8 minutes

Servings: 8

Size/ Portion: 1 slice

Ingredients

- 1 (9-inch) prepared graham cracker crust
- 3 cups of sweetened condensed milk
- 1/2 cup sour cream
- 3/4 cup lime juice
- 1 tablespoon grated lime zest

Direction

1. Prepare oven to 175 ° C
2. Combine the condensed milk, sour cream, lime juice, and lime zest in a medium bowl. Mix well and pour into the graham cracker crust.
3. Bake in the preheated oven for 5 to 8 minutes
4. Cool the cake well before serving. Decorate with lime slices and whipped cream if desired.

Nutrition: 553 calories 20.5g fat 10.9g protein

Rhubarb Strawberry Crunch

Preparation Time: 15 minutes

Cooking Time: 45 minutes

Servings: 18

Size/ Portion: 1 cup

Ingredients

- 1 cup of white sugar
- 3 tablespoons all-purpose flour
- 3 cups of fresh strawberries, sliced
- 3 cups of rhubarb, cut into cubes
- 1 1/2 cup flour
- 1 cup packed brown sugar
- 1 cup butter
- 1 cup oatmeal

Direction

1. Preheat the oven to 190 ° C.
2. Combine white sugar, 3 tablespoons flour, strawberries and rhubarb in a large bowl. Place the mixture in a 9 x 13-inch baking dish.
3. Mix 1 1/2 cups of flour, brown sugar, butter, and oats until a crumbly texture is obtained. You may want to use a blender for this. Crumble the mixture of rhubarb and strawberry.

4. Bake for 45 minutes.

Nutrition: 253 calories 10.8g fat 2.3g protein

Chocolate Chip Banana Dessert

Preparation Time: 20 minutes

Cooking Time: 20 minutes

Servings: 24

Size/ Portion:

Ingredients

- 2/3 cup white sugar
- 3/4 cup butter
- 2/3 cup brown sugar
- 1 egg, beaten slightly
- 1 teaspoon vanilla extract
- 1 cup of banana puree
- 1 3/4 cup flour
- 2 teaspoons baking powder
- 1/2 teaspoon of salt
- 1 cup of semi-sweet chocolate chips

Direction:

1. Ready the oven to 175 ° C Grease and bake a 10 x 15-inch baking pan.
2. Beat the butter, white sugar, and brown sugar in a large bowl until light. Beat the egg and vanilla. Fold in the banana puree: mix baking powder, flour, and

salt in another bowl. Mix flour mixture into the butter mixture. Stir in the chocolate chips. Spread in pan.

3. Bake for 20 minutes. Cool before cutting into squares.

Nutrition: 174 calories 8.2g fat 1.7g protein

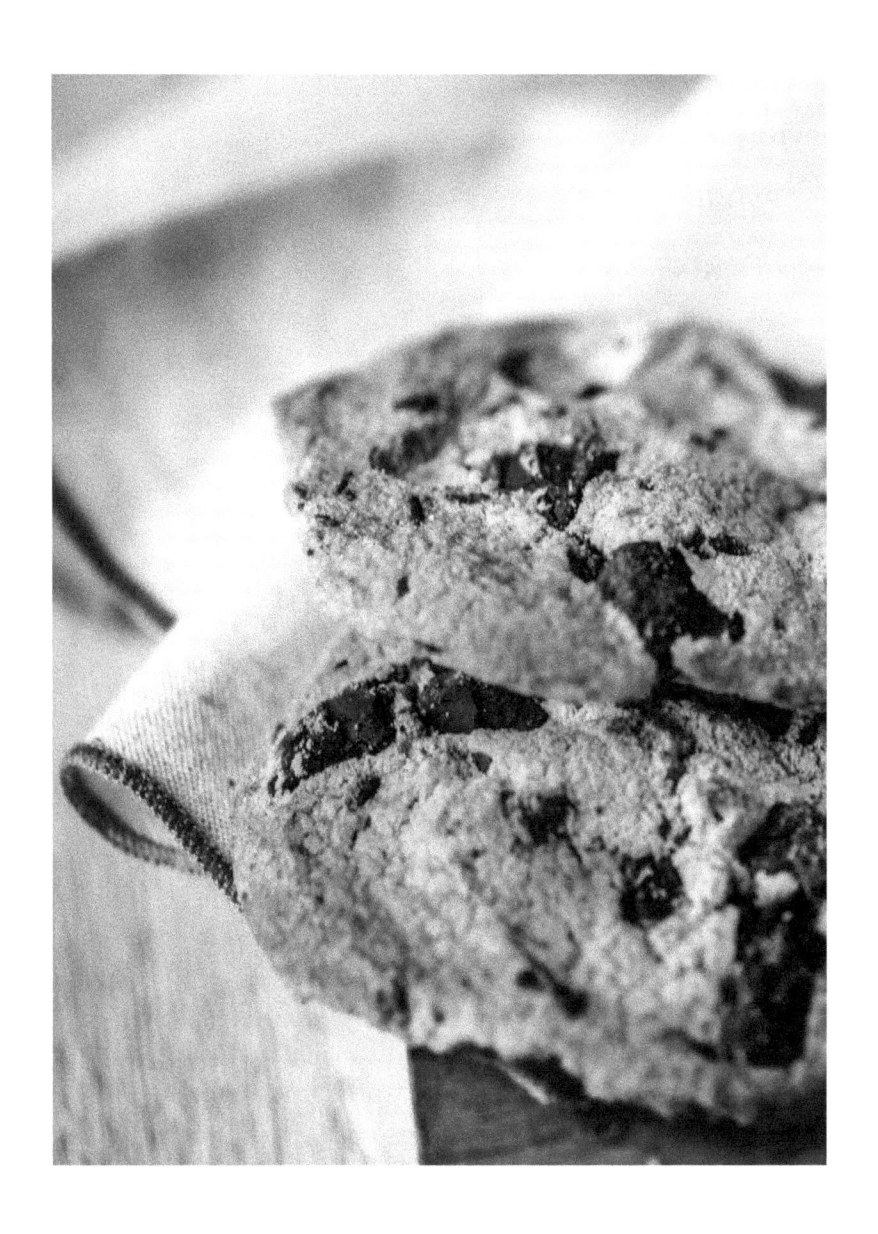

Apple Pie Filling

Preparation Time: 20 minutes

Cooking Time: 12 minutes

Servings: 40

Size/ Portion: 1 cup

Ingredients

- 18 cups chopped apples
- 3 tablespoons lemon juice
- 10 cups of water
- 4 1/2 cups of white sugar
- 1 cup corn flour
- 2 teaspoons of ground cinnamon
- 1 teaspoon of salt
- 1/4 teaspoon ground nutmeg

Direction

1. Mix apples with lemon juice in a large bowl and set aside. Pour the water in a Dutch oven over medium heat. Combine sugar, corn flour, cinnamon, salt, and nutmeg in a bowl. Add to water, mix well, and bring to a boil. Cook for 2 minutes with continuous stirring.

2. Boil apples again. Reduce the heat, cover, and simmer for 8 minutes. Allow cooling for 30 minutes.

3. Pour into five freezer containers and leave 1/2 inch of free space. Cool to room temperature.

4. Seal and freeze

Nutrition: 129 calories 0.1g fat 0.2g protein

Ice Cream Sandwich Dessert

Preparation Time: 20 minutes

Cooking Time: 0 minute

Servings: 12

Size/ Portion: 2 squares

Ingredients

- 22 ice cream sandwiches
- Frozen whipped topping in 16 oz. container, thawed
- 1 jar (12 oz.) Caramel ice cream
- 1 1/2 cups of salted peanuts

Direction

1. Cut a sandwich with ice in two. Place a whole sandwich and a half sandwich on a short side of a 9 x 13-inch baking dish. Repeat this until the bottom is covered, alternate the full sandwich, and the half sandwich.
2. Spread half of the whipped topping. Pour the caramel over it. Sprinkle with half the peanuts. Do layers with the rest of the ice cream sandwiches, whipped cream, and peanuts.
3. Cover and freeze for up to 2 months. Remove from the freezer 20 minutes before serving. Cut into squares.

Nutrition: 559 calories 28.8g fat 10g protein

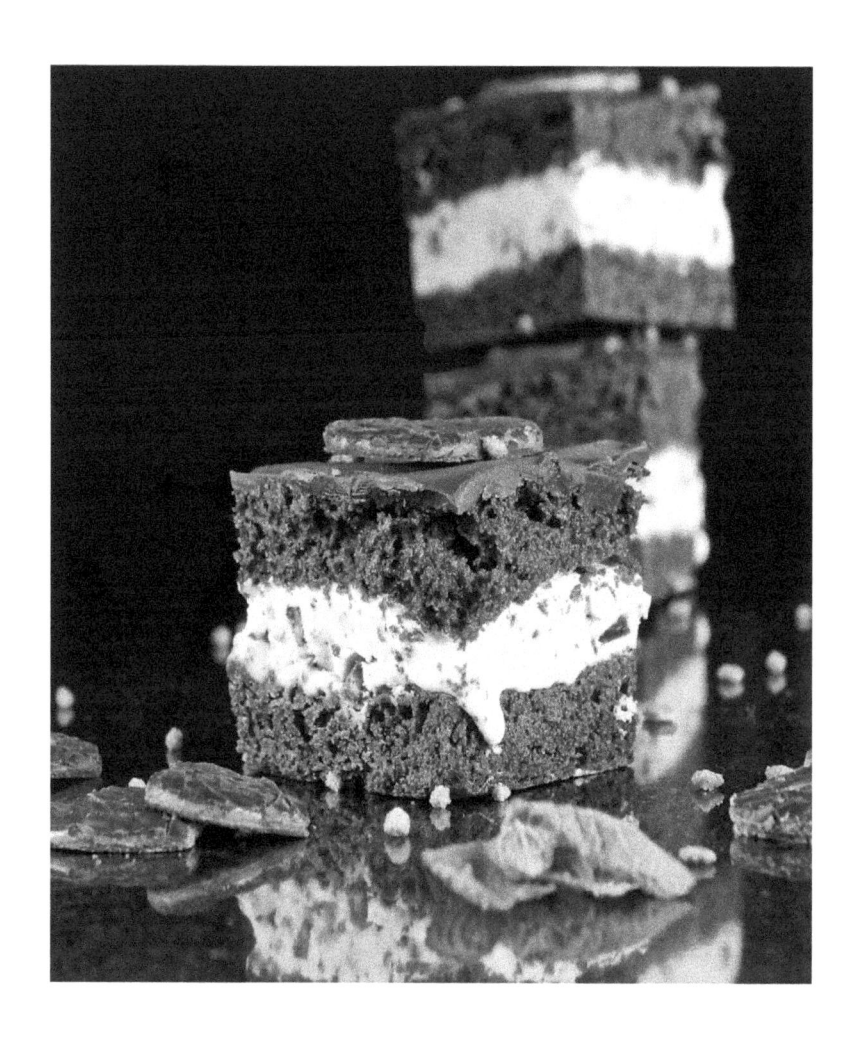

Cranberry and Pistachio Biscotti

Preparation Time: 15 minutes

Cooking Time: 35 minutes

Servings: 36

Size/ Portion: 2 slices

Ingredients

- 1/4 cup light olive oil
- 3/4 cup white sugar
- 2 teaspoons vanilla extract
- 1/2 teaspoon almond extract
- 2 eggs
- 1 3/4 cup all-purpose flour
- 1/4 teaspoon salt
- 1 teaspoon baking powder
- 1/2 cup dried cranberries
- 1 1/2 cup pistachio nuts

Direction

1. Prep oven to 150 ° C
2. Combine the oil and sugar in a large bowl until a homogeneous mixture is obtained. Stir in the vanilla and almond extract and add the eggs. Combine flour,

salt, and baking powder; gradually add to the egg mixture — mix cranberries and nuts by hand.

3. Divide the dough in half — form two 12 x 2-inch logs on a parchment baking sheet. The dough can be sticky, wet hands with cold water to make it easier to handle the dough.

4. Bake in the preheated oven for 35 minutes or until the blocks are golden brown. Pullout from the oven and let cool for 10 minutes. Reduce oven heat to 275 degrees F (135 degrees C).

5. Cut diagonally into 3/4-inch-thick slices. Place on the sides on the baking sheet covered with parchment — Bake for about 8 to 10 minutes

Nutrition: 92 calories 4.3g fat 2.1g protein

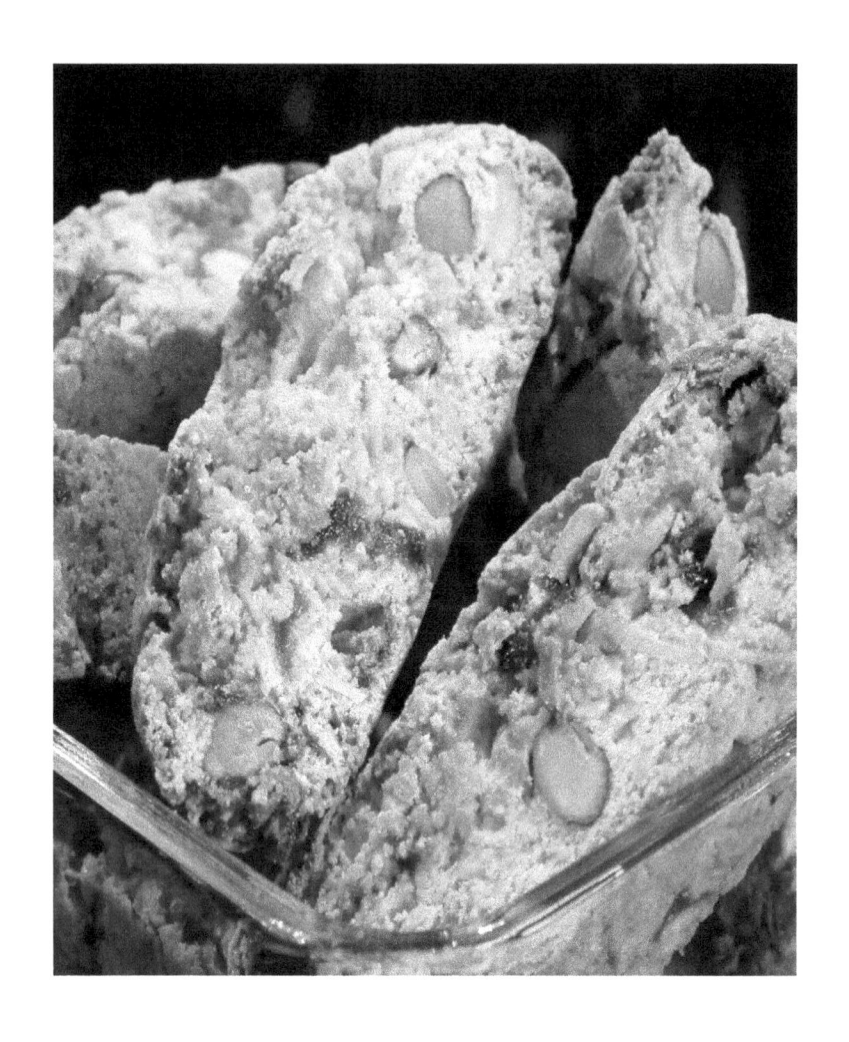

Cream Puff Dessert

Preparation Time: 20 minutes

Cooking Time: 36 minutes

Servings: 12

Size/ Portion: 2 puffs

Ingredients

Puff

- 1 cup water
- 1/2 cup butter
- 1 cup all-purpose flour
- 4 eggs

Filling

- 1 (8-oz) package cream cheese, softened
- 3 1/2 cups cold milk
- 2 (4-oz) packages instant chocolate pudding mix

Topping

- 1 (8-oz) package frozen whipped cream topping, thawed
- 1/4 cup topping with milk chocolate flavor
- 1/4 cup caramel filling
- 1/3 cup almond flakes

Direction:

1. Set oven to 200 degrees C (400 degrees F). Grease a 9 x 13-inch baking dish.

2. Melt the butter in the water in a medium-sized pan over medium heat. Pour the flour in one go and mix vigorously until the mixture forms a ball. Remove from heat and let stand for 5 minutes. Beat the eggs one by one until they are smooth and shiny. Spread in the prepared pan.

3. Bake in the preheated oven for 30 to 35 minutes, until puffed and browned. Cool completely on a rack.

4. While the puff pastry cools, mix the cream cheese mixture, the milk, and the pudding. Spread over the cooled puff pastry. Cool for 20 minutes.

5. Spread whipped cream on cooled topping and sprinkle with chocolate and caramel sauce. Sprinkle with almonds. Freeze 1 hour before serving.

Nutrition: 355 calories 22.3g fat 8.7g protein

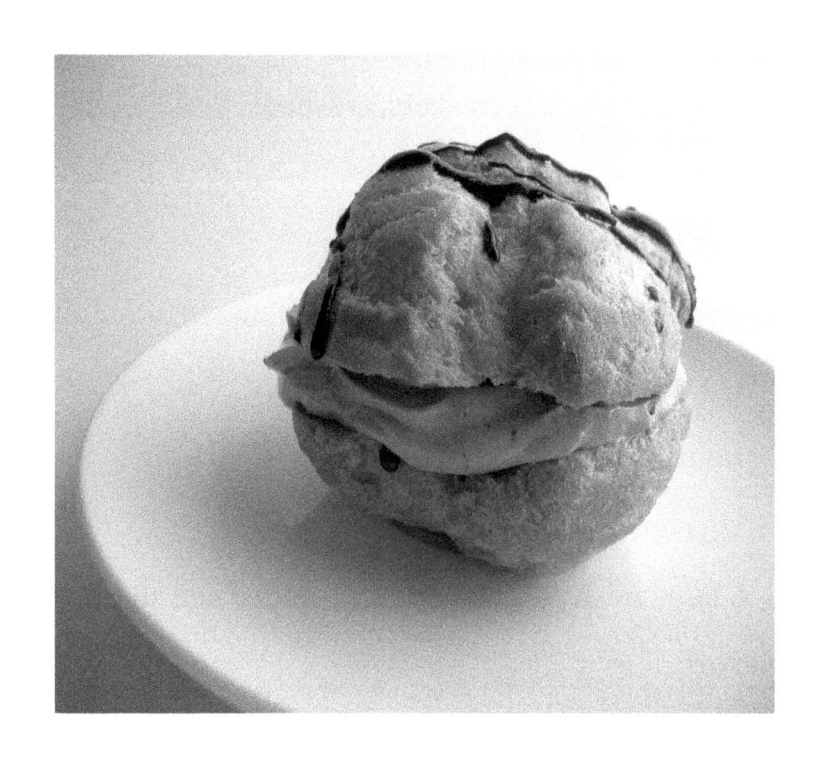

Fresh Peach Dessert

Preparation Time: 30 minutes

Cooking Time: 27 minutes

Servings: 15

Size/ portion: 1 cup

Ingredients

- 16 whole graham crackers, crushed
- 3/4 cup melted butter
- 1/2 cup white sugar
- 4 1/2 cups of miniature marshmallows
- 1/4 cup of milk
- 1 pint of heavy cream
- 1/3 cup of white sugar
- 6 large fresh peaches - peeled, seeded and sliced

Direction:

1. In a bowl, mix the crumbs from the graham cracker, melted butter, and 1/2 cup of sugar. Mix until a homogeneous mixture is obtained, save 1/4 cup of the mixture for filling. Squeeze the rest of the mixture into the bottom of a 9 x 13-inch baking dish.

2. Heat marshmallows and milk in a large pan over low heat and stir until marshmallows are completely melted. Remove from heat and let cool.

3. Beat the cream in a large bowl until soft peaks occur. Beat 1/3 cup of sugar until the cream forms firm spikes. Add the whipped cream to the cooled marshmallow mixture.

4. Divide half of the cream mixture over the crust, place the peaches over the cream and divide the rest of the cream mixture over the peaches. Sprinkle the crumb mixture on the cream. Cool until ready to serve.

Nutrition: 366 calories 22.5g fat 1.9g protein

Blueberry Dessert

Preparation Time: 30 minutes

Cooking Time: 20 minutes

Servings: 28

Size/ Portion: 1 slice

Ingredients

- 1/2 cup butter
- 2 cups white sugar
- 36 graham crackers, crushed
- 4 eggs
- 2 packets of cream cheese, softened
- 1 teaspoon vanilla extract
- 2 cans of blueberry pie filling
- 1 package (16-oz) frozen whipped cream, thawed

Direction:

1. Cook butter and sprinkle 1 cup of sugar and graham crackers. Squeeze this mixture into a 9x13 dish.
2. Beat the eggs. Gradually beat the cream cheese, sugar, and vanilla in the eggs.
3. Pour the mixture of eggs and cream cheese over the graham cracker crust. Bake for 15 to 20 minutes at 165 ° C (325 ° F). Cool.

4. Pour the blueberry pie filling on top of the baked dessert. Spread non-dairy whipped topping on fruit. Cool until ready to serve.

Nutrition: 354 calories 15.4g fat 3.8g protein

Good Sweet

Preparation Time: 10 minutes

Cooking Time: 10 minutes

Servings: 2

Size/ Portion: 1 cup

Ingredients:

- Tomatoes, ¼ teaspoon, chopped
- Cucumber, ¼ teaspoon, chopped
- Honey, 2 tablespoons
- Other veggies/beans optional

Directions:

1. Whisk the ingredients well.
2. In a bowl, toss to coat with honey as smoothly as possible.

Nutrition: 187 Calories 15.6g Fat 2g Protein

A Taste of Dessert

Preparation Time: 15 minutes

Cooking Time: 0 minutes

Servings: 2

Size/ Portion: 1 bowl

Ingredients:

- Cilantro, 1 tablespoon
- Green onion, 1 tablespoon
- Mango, 1 peeled, seeded and chopped
- Bell pepper, ¼ cup, chopped
- Honey, 2 tablespoons

Directions:
1. Incorporate all the ingredients.
2. Serve when combined well.

Nutrition: 21 Calories 0.1g Fat 0.3g Protein

Honey Carrots

Preparation Time: 5 minutes

Cooking Time: 15 minutes

Servings: 2

Size/ portion: 8 ounces

Ingredients:

- Baby carrots, 16 ounces
- Brown sugar, ¼ cup

Directions:

1. Boil carrots with water in a huge pot
2. Drain after 15 minutes, and steam for 2 minutes.
3. Stir in the sugar, and serve when mixed well.

Nutrition: 402 Calories 23.3g Fat 1.4g Protein

Fresh Cherry Treat

Preparation Time: 10 minutes

Cooking Time: 10 minutes

Servings: 2

Size/ Portion: 2 ounces

Ingredients:

- Honey, 1 tablespoon
- Almonds, 1 tablespoon, crushed
- Cherries, 12 ounces

Directions:

1. Preheat the oven to 350F, and for 5 minutes, bake the cherries.
2. Coat them with honey, and serve with almonds on top.

Nutrition: 448 Calories 36.4g Fat 3.5g Protein

Milky Peachy Dessert

Preparation Time: 15 minutes

Cooking Time: 10 minutes

Servings: 2

Size/ Portion: 1 cup

Ingredients:

- Peach, 1 fresh, peeled and sliced
- Brown sugar, 1 teaspoon
- Milk, 1 tablespoon

Directions:

1. Prepare a baking dish with a layer of peaches and toss in the milk.
2. Top the peaches with sugar, and bake at 350F for 5 minutes.

Nutrition: 366 Calories 22.5g Fat 1.9g Protein

Citrus Sections

Preparation Time: 20 minutes

Cooking Time: 5 minutes

Servings: 2

Size/ Portion: 2 section

Ingredients:

- Grapefruit, 1, peeled and sectioned
- Pineapple, ½ cup, chunks
- Oranges, 1 small, sectioned into chunks
- Brown sugar, ½ tablespoon
- Butter, low fat and unsalted, ½ teaspoon, melted

Directions:

1. Preheat an oven tray at 350F.
2. Set the fruits on the tray, and top with the brown sugar, mixed with the butter, and bake for 5 minutes.
3. Transfer to a platter.

Nutrition: 279 Calories 5.9g Fat 2.2g Protein

After Meal Apples

Preparation Time: 15 minutes

Cooking Time: 25 minutes

Servings: 2

Size/ Portion: 1 piece

Ingredients:

- Apple, 1 whole, cut into chunks
- Pineapple chunks, ½ cups
- Grapes, seedless, ½ cup
- Orange juice, ¼ cup
- Cinnamon, ¼ teaspoon

Directions:

1. Preheat the oven to 350F.
2. Add all the fruits to a baking dish.
3. Drizzle with the orange juice and sprinkle with cinnamon.
4. Bake for 25 minutes, and serve hot.

Nutrition: 124 Calories 3.2g Fat 0.8g Protein

Warm Nut Bites

Preparation Time: 10 minutes

Cooking Time: 20 minutes

Servings: 2

Size/ Portion 2 bites

Ingredients:

- Honey, 4 tablespoons
- Almonds, 2 cups
- Almond oil, 1 tablespoon

Directions:

1. Layer the almonds, whole, on a baking sheet.
2. Bake for 15 minutes at 350F.
3. Turn half way, and roll the almonds in honey.
4. Serve.

Nutrition: 268 Calories 19.7g Fat 7.6g Protein

Dipped Sprouts

Preparation Time: 12 minutes

Cooking Time: 10 minutes

Servings: 2

Size/ portion: 4 ounces

Ingredients:

- Brussels sprouts, 16 ounces
- Honey, 4 tablespoons
- Raisins and nuts, crushed, 6 tablespoons

Directions:

1. Boil water in a pot.
2. Add sprouts, and cook for 10 minutes until soft.
2. Glaze the sprouts in honey, and coat well. Add nuts and raisins.

Nutrition: 221 Calories 15.1g Fat 5.3g Protein

Pecans and Cheese

Preparation Time: 20 minutes

Cooking Time: 0 minutes

Servings: 2

Size/ Portion: 3 ounces

Ingredients:

- Cinnamon, ground, 1 teaspoon
- Feta cheese, 4 ounces
- Pecans, finely chopped, 2 ounces
- Honey, 2 tablespoons
- Rosemary, fresh, 2 sprigs, minced

Directions:

1. Make small balls of the cheese.
3. Crush the pecans and place them in a shallow bowl with the cinnamon.
4. Roll the cheese in the pecans and cinnamon.
5. Drizzle honey over the balls.
6. Serve with rosemary on top.

Nutrition: 234 Calories 18.6g Fat 7.5g Protein

Hazelnut Cookies

Preparation Time: 8 minutes

Cooking Time: 21 minutes

Servings: 5

Size/ portion: 2 cookies

Ingredients:

- 1 1/4 cups hazelnut meal
- 6 tbsp. flour
- 1 tbsp. brown sugar
- 2 tbsp. powdered sugar
- 1/2 tsp. kosher salt
- 1/2 lemon zest
- 1/2 lemon juice
- 1/2 tsp. vanilla
- 1/4 cup extra virgin olive oil

Directions:

1. Heat the oven at 375 degrees F.
2. Take a bowl, add the hazelnut meal, brown sugar, flour, half of the powdered sugar, lemon zest, and salt. Next, whisk it well.
3. Whisk olive oil and vanilla.
4. Once the dough is crumbly, shape them into cookies and line them on the baking sheet.

5. Bake it until the edges are lightly brown, around 20 minutes.
7. Take out on a cooling rack Let it sit to cool.
8. Meanwhile, take a small bowl and add lemon juice, and the remaining powdered sugar.
9. Drizzle the syrup over the cookies before serving.

Nutrition: 276 Calories 3.6g Protein 21.2g Fat

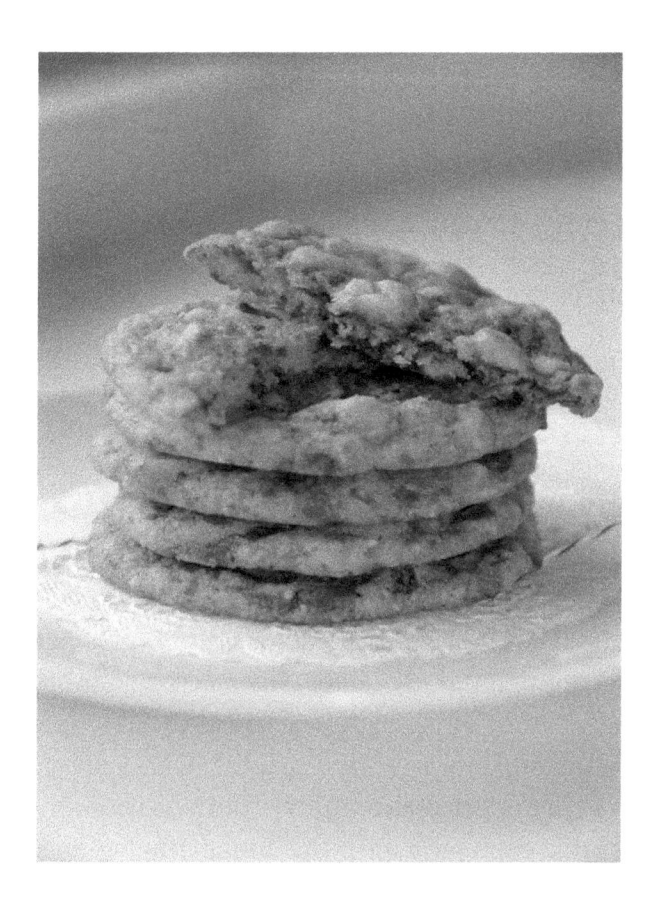

Fruit Dessert Nachos

Preparation Time: 9 minutes

Cooking Time: 13 minutes

Servings: 3

Size/ Portion: 2 pieces

Ingredients:

- 1 tbsp. sugar
- a pinch of ground cinnamon
- 1 1/2 whole wheat tortillas
- 1/4 cup softened light cream cheese
- 1 cup chopped assorted melon
- 2 1/2 tbsp. light dairy sour cream
- 1/2 tsp. finely shredded orange peel
- 1 tbsp. orange juice

Directions:

1. Preheat oven at 425 degrees F.
2. Grease huge baking sheet with cooking spray.
3. Take a small bowl, combine the cinnamon and half of the sugar.
4. Take the tortillas and lightly coat with cooking spray. Sprinkle each side with the sugar mix.
5. Cut the tortillas to make 8 wedges and place them on the baking sheet.

6. Bake the tortillas until they turn light browned, for about 7 to 8 minutes. Turn once halfway.
7. Meanwhile, take a small sized bowl and mix together the sour cream, cream cheese, 30 grams of orange juice, orange peel and the remaining sugar. Once smooth, set it aside.
8. Take a medium bowl and combine together melon and remaining orange juice.
10. Serve by adding a spoon of melon mix on each tortilla wedge, and a spoon of cream cheese mixture.

Nutrition: 121 Calories 5.3g Protein 5.2g Fat

Honey Yogurt with Berries

Preparation Time: 12 minutes

Cooking Time: 0 minute

Servings: 2

Size/ Portion: 1 cup

Ingredients:

- 4 oz. hulled, halved strawberries
- 1/6 cup Greek yogurt
- 1/2 cup blueberries
- 1/2 cup raspberries
- 1 tsp. honey
- 1/2 tbsp. balsamic vinegar

Directions:

1. Take a large bowl and toss the berries with the balsamic vinegar.
2. Set it aside for 8 to 10 minutes.
3. Meanwhile, mix together the honey and yogurt in a bowl.
4. Serve it by topping the berries with honey yogurt.

Nutrition: 111 Calories 4.6g Protein 3g Fat

Lightning Source UK Ltd.
Milton Keynes UK
UKHW021846080121
376714UK00003B/271